LYMPHEDEMA DIET

MAIN COURSE - 60+ Breakfast, Lunch, Dinner and Dessert Recipes for Lymphedema Diet

TABLE OF CONTENTS

BREAKFAST 7

COCONUT PANCAKES 7

GOJI BERRIES PANCAKES 9

KIWI PANCAKES 10

MANGO PANCAKES 11

SIMPLE PANCAKES 12

GINGERBREAD MUFFINS 13

PEAR MUFFINS 15

POMELO MUFFINS 17

APPLE MUFFINS 19

CHOCOLATE MUFFINS 21

SIMPLE MUFFINS 23

SPINACH OMELETTE 25

CUCUMBER OMELETTE 27

BASIL OMELETTE 29

CHEESE OMELETTE 31

OLIVE OMELETTE 33

AVOCADO TOAST 35

BREAKFAST POTATOES 36

BREAKFAST CASSEROLE 37

TAQUITOS 39

LUNCH 42

CAULIFLOWER RECIPE 42

BROCCOLI RECIPE 44

TOMATOES & HAM PIZZA 45

CAULIFLOWER SOUP 47

GARLIC SOUP 49

LEEK SOUP 51

CARROT SOUP 53

CELERY SOUP 55

ASPARAGUS FRITATTA 57

CORN FRITATTA 59

EDAMAME FRITATTA 61

PROSCIUTTO FRITATTA 63

EGGPLANT FRITATTA 65

SWEET POTATO FRIES 67

ROASTED CHICKPEAS 68

CHEESE ROLLS 69

BAKED SALMON 71

GARLIC PASTA 72

CRANBERRY PECAN SALAD 74

PEAR SALAD 75

WATERMELON SALAD 76

POTATO SALAD 77

SOUTHWESTERN SALAD 78

TOMATO SALAD 79

MELON SALAD 80

CAPRESE SALAD 81

KIWI SALAD 82

KALE SALAD 83

DINNER 85

SIMPLE PIZZA RECIPE 85

ZUCCHINI PIZZA 87

SMOOTHIES 89

SUMMER SMOOTHIE 89

GREEN SMOOTHIE 90

TROPICAL SMOOTHIE 91

BERRY SMOOTHIE 92

CITRUS SMOOTHIE 93

POMEGRANATE SMOOTHIE 94

PEANUT BUTTER SMOOTHIE 95

MANGO SMOOTHIE 96

START YOUR DAY SMOOTHIE 97

PAPAYA SMOOTHIE 98

purposes solely, and is universal as so. The presentation of the information is without contract or any type of guarantee assurance.

The trademarks that are used are without any consent, and the publication of the trademark is without permission or backing by the trademark owner. All trademarks and brands within this book are for clarifying purposes only and are the owned by the owners themselves, not affiliated with this document.

Introduction

Lymphedema recipes for personal enjoyment but also for family enjoyment. You will love them for sure for how easy it is to prepare them.

COCONUT PANCAKES

Serves: *4*

Prep Time: *10*   Minutes

Cook Time: *20*   Minutes

Total Time: *30*   Minutes

INGREDIENTS

- 1 cup whole wheat flour
- ¼ tsp baking soda
- ¼ tsp baking powder
- 1 cup coconut flakes
- 2 eggs
- 1 cup milk

DIRECTIONS

1. In a bowl combine all ingredients together and mix well
2. In a skillet heat olive oil

3. Pour ¼ of the batter and cook each pancake for 1-2 minutes per side

4. When ready remove from heat and serve

Serves: **4**

Prep Time: **10**   Minutes

Cook Time: **30**   Minutes

Total Time: **40**   Minutes

INGREDIENTS

- 1 cup whole wheat flour
- ¼ tsp baking soda
- ¼ tsp baking powder
- 2 tablespoons goji berries
- 2 eggs
- 1 cup milk

DIRECTIONS

1. In a bowl combine all ingredients together and mix well
2. In a skillet heat olive oil
3. Pour ¼ of the batter and cook each pancake for 1-2 minutes per side
4. When ready remove from heat and serve

Serves: **4**

Prep Time: **10** Minutes

Cook Time: **20** Minutes

Total Time: **30** Minutes

INGREDIENTS

- 1 cup whole wheat flour
- ¼ tsp baking soda
- ¼ tsp baking powder
- 1 cup mashed kiwi
- 2 eggs
- 1 cup milk

DIRECTIONS

1. In a bowl combine all ingredients together and mix well
2. In a skillet heat olive oil
3. Pour ¼ of the batter and cook each pancake for 1-2 minutes per side
4. When ready remove from heat and serve

Serves: **4**

Prep Time: **10**   Minutes

Cook Time: **20**   Minutes

Total Time: **30**   Minutes

INGREDIENTS

- 1 cup whole wheat flour
- ¼ tsp baking soda
- ¼ tsp baking powder
- 1 cup mashed mango
- 2 eggs
- 1 cup milk

DIRECTIONS

1. In a bowl combine all ingredients together and mix well
2. In a skillet heat olive oil
3. Pour ¼ of the batter and cook each pancake for 1-2 minutes per side
4. When ready remove from heat and serve

Serves: *4*
Prep Time: *10*   Minutes

Cook Time: *30*   Minutes

Total Time: *40*   Minutes

INGREDIENTS

- 1 cup whole wheat flour
- ¼ tsp baking soda
- ¼ tsp baking powder
- 2 eggs
- 1 cup milk

DIRECTIONS

1. In a bowl combine all ingredients together and mix well
2. In a skillet heat olive oil
3. Pour ¼ of the batter and cook each pancake for 1-2 minutes per side
4. When ready remove from heat and serve

Serves:	*8-12*	
Prep Time:	*10*	Minutes
Cook Time:	*20*	Minutes
Total Time:	*30*	Minutes

INGREDIENTS

- 2 eggs
- 1 tablespoon olive oil
- 1 cup milk
- 2 cups whole wheat flour
- 1 tsp baking soda
- ¼ tsp baking soda
- 1 tsp ginger
- 1 tsp cinnamon
- ¼ cup molasses

DIRECTIONS

1. In a bowl combine all dry ingredients
2. In another bowl combine all dry ingredients

3. Combine wet and dry ingredients together

4. Fold in ginger and mix well

5. Pour mixture into 8-12 prepared muffin cups, fill 2/3 of the cups

6. Bake for 18-20 minutes at 375 F

7. When ready remove from the oven and serve

Serves: **8-12**

Prep Time: **10** Minutes

Cook Time: **20** Minutes

Total Time: **30** Minutes

INGREDIENTS

- 2 eggs
- 1 tablespoon olive oil
- 1 cup milk
- 2 cups whole wheat flour
- 1 tsp baking soda
- ¼ tsp baking soda
- 1 tsp cinnamon
- 1 cup mashed pear

DIRECTIONS

1. In a bowl combine all dry ingredients
2. In another bowl combine all dry ingredients
3. Combine wet and dry ingredients together

4. Pour mixture into 8-12 prepared muffin cups, fill 2/3 of the cups

5. Bake for 18-20 minutes at 375 F

6. When ready remove from the oven and serve

Serves: **8-12**
Prep Time: **10**   Minutes

Cook Time: **20**   Minutes

Total Time: **30**   Minutes

INGREDIENTS

- 2 eggs
- 1 tablespoon olive oil
- 1 cup milk
- 2 cups whole wheat flour
- 1 tsp baking soda
- ¼ tsp baking soda
- 1 tsp cinnamon
- 1 cup pomelo

DIRECTIONS

1. In a bowl combine all dry ingredients
2. In another bowl combine all dry ingredients
3. Combine wet and dry ingredients together

4. Pour mixture into 8-12 prepared muffin cups, fill
    2/3 of the cups

5. Bake for 18-20 minutes at 375 F

6. When ready remove from the oven and serve

Serves: *8-12*

Prep Time: *10*   Minutes

Cook Time: *20*   Minutes

Total Time: *30*   Minutes

INGREDIENTS

- 2 eggs
- 1 tablespoon olive oil
- 1 cup milk
- 2 cups whole wheat flour
- 1 tsp baking soda
- ¼ tsp baking soda
- 1 tsp cinnamon
- 1 cup apple

DIRECTIONS

1. In a bowl combine all dry ingredients
2. In another bowl combine all dry ingredients
3. Combine wet and dry ingredients together

4. Pour mixture into 8-12 prepared muffin cups, fill
   2/3 of the cups

5. Bake for 18-20 minutes at 375 F

6. When ready remove from the oven and serve

Serves: *8-12*
Prep Time: *10*   Minutes

Cook Time: *20*   Minutes

Total Time: *30*   Minutes

INGREDIENTS

- 2 eggs
- 1 tablespoon olive oil
- 1 cup milk
- 2 cups whole wheat flour
- 1 tsp baking soda
- ¼ tsp baking soda
- 1 tsp cinnamon
- 1 cup chocolate chips

DIRECTIONS

1. In a bowl combine all dry ingredients
2. In another bowl combine all dry ingredients
3. Combine wet and dry ingredients together

4. Fold in chocolate chips and mix well

5. Pour mixture into 8-12 prepared muffin cups, fill 2/3 of the cups

6. Bake for 18-20 minutes at 375 F

7. When ready remove from the oven and serve

Serves: **8-12**

Prep Time: **10** Minutes

Cook Time: **20** Minutes

Total Time: **30** Minutes

INGREDIENTS

- 2 eggs
- 1 tablespoon olive oil
- 1 cup milk
- 2 cups whole wheat flour
- 1 tsp baking soda
- ¼ tsp baking soda
- 1 tsp cinnamon

DIRECTIONS

1. In a bowl combine all dry ingredients
2. In another bowl combine all dry ingredients
3. Combine wet and dry ingredients together

4. Pour mixture into 8-12 prepared muffin cups, fill 2/3 of the cups

5. Bake for 18-20 minutes at 375 F

6. When ready remove from the oven and serve

Serves: *1*
Prep Time: *5* Minutes

Cook Time: *10* Minutes

Total Time: *15* Minutes

INGREDIENTS

- 2 eggs
- ¼ tsp salt
- ¼ tsp black pepper
- 1 tablespoon olive oil
- ¼ cup cheese
- ¼ tsp basil
- 1 cup spinach

DIRECTIONS

1. In a bowl combine all ingredients together and mix well
2. In a skillet heat olive oil and pour the egg mixture
3. Cook for 1-2 minutes per side

4. When ready remove omelette from the skillet and
    serve

Serves: *1*
Prep Time: *5*   Minutes

Cook Time: *10*   Minutes

Total Time: *15*   Minutes

INGREDIENTS

- **2 eggs**
- **¼ tsp salt**
- **¼ tsp black pepper**
- **1 tablespoon olive oil**
- **¼ cup cheese**
- **¼ tsp basil**
- **½ cup cucumber**

DIRECTIONS

1. **In a bowl combine all ingredients together and mix well**
2. **In a skillet heat olive oil and pour the egg mixture**
3. **Cook for 1-2 minutes per side**

4. When ready remove omelette from the skillet and
    serve

Serves: *1*
Prep Time: *5*   Minutes

Cook Time: *10*   Minutes

Total Time: *15*   Minutes

INGREDIENTS

- **2 eggs**
- **¼ tsp salt**
- **¼ tsp black pepper**
- **1 tablespoon olive oil**
- **¼ cup cheese**
- **¼ tsp basil**
- **1 cup red onion**

DIRECTIONS

1. **In a bowl combine all ingredients together and mix well**
2. **In a skillet heat olive oil and pour the egg mixture**
3. **Cook for 1-2 minutes per side**

4. When ready remove omelette from the skillet and
    serve

Serves: *1*

Prep Time: *5* Minutes

Cook Time: *10* Minutes

Total Time: *15* Minutes

INGREDIENTS

- 2 eggs
- ¼ tsp salt
- ¼ tsp black pepper
- 1 tablespoon olive oil
- ¼ cup cheese
- ¼ tsp basil
- 1 cup mushrooms

DIRECTIONS

1. In a bowl combine all ingredients together and mix well
2. In a skillet heat olive oil and pour the egg mixture
3. Cook for 1-2 minutes per side

4. **When ready remove omelette from the skillet and
    serve**

Serves: *1*

Prep Time: *5*   Minutes

Cook Time: *10*   Minutes

Total Time: *15*   Minutes

INGREDIENTS

- 2 eggs
- ¼ tsp salt
- ¼ tsp black pepper
- 1 tablespoon olive oil
- ¼ cup cheese
- ¼ cup Kalamata olives
- ¼ tsp basil
- 1 cup tomatoes

DIRECTIONS

1. In a bowl combine all ingredients together and mix well

2. In a skillet heat olive oil and pour the egg mixture

3. Cook for 1-2 minutes per side

4. When ready remove omelette from the skillet and
    serve

Serves: 2
Prep Time: 5   Minutes

Cook Time: 5   Minutes

Total Time: *10*   Minutes

INGREDIENTS

- 2 slices bread
- ½ avocado
- 2 tablespoons hemp seeds
- ¼ tsp pepper

DIRECTIONS

1. Toast the bread slices
2. Mass the avocado and spread on the bread
3. Top with hemp seeds and a dash of pepper
4. Serve when ready

Serves: *4*
Prep Time: *10* Minutes

Cook Time: *20* Minutes

Total Time: *30* Minutes

INGREDIENTS

- 2 potatoes
- 2 tablespoons olive oil
- 1 pinch salt
- 1 tablespoon parmesan cheese

DIRECTIONS

1. In a skillet heat olive oil
2. Add slices of potatoes and fry on low heat
3. Sprinkle with salt and cook until the potatoes are brown
4. When ready transfer to a plate, sprinkle parmesan cheese and serve

Serves: *4*

Prep Time: *10* Minutes

Cook Time: *35* Minutes

Total Time: *45* Minutes

INGREDIENTS

- 1 can crescent rolls
- 1 lb. bacon
- 1 cup cheddar cheese
- 4 eggs
- ¼ cup almond milk
- ¼ tsp salt

DIRECTIONS

1. Sprinkle bacon and cheese
2. In a bowl whisk eggs and milk together
3. Pour mixture over the cheese mixture
4. Bake at 350 F for 28-30 minutes

5. When ready remove from heat and serve

38

Serves: **8-10**
Prep Time: **10**   Minutes

Cook Time: **20**   Minutes

Total Time: **30**   Minutes

INGREDIENTS

- 8-10 corn tortillas
- 4 eggs
- 7-8 oz. sausage
- ½ cup tomatoes
- 1 avocado
- 1 cup cheddar cheese

DIRECTIONS

1. Scramble the eggs and place them on each tortilla
2. Add sausage, tomatoes, avocado and cheddar cheese
3. Roll and place the tortillas on a baking sheet
4. Bake at 400 F for 15-18 minutes

5. When ready remove from heat and serve

CAULIFLOWER RECIPE

Serves: **6-8**

Prep Time: **10**   Minutes

Cook Time: **15**   Minutes

Total Time: **25**   Minutes

INGREDIENTS

- 1 pizza crust
- ½ cup tomato sauce
- ¼ black pepper
- 1 cup cauliflower
- 1 cup mozzarella cheese
- 1 cup olives

DIRECTIONS

1. Spread tomato sauce on the pizza crust
2. Place all the toppings on the pizza crust
3. Bake the pizza at 425 F for 12-15 minutes

4. When ready remove pizza from the oven and
    serve

Serves: *6-8*
Prep Time: *10*   Minutes

Cook Time: *15*   Minutes

Total Time: *25*   Minutes

INGREDIENTS

- 1 pizza crust
- ½ cup tomato sauce
- ¼ black pepper
- 1 cup broccoli
- 1 cup mozzarella cheese
- 1 cup olives

DIRECTIONS

1. Spread tomato sauce on the pizza crust
2. Place all the toppings on the pizza crust
3. Bake the pizza at 425 F for 12-15 minutes
4. When ready remove pizza from the oven and serve

Serves: *6-8*

Prep Time: *10* Minutes

Cook Time: *15* Minutes

Total Time: *25* Minutes

INGREDIENTS

- 1 pizza crust
- ½ cup tomato sauce
- ¼ black pepper
- 1 cup pepperoni slices
- 1 cup tomatoes
- 6-8 ham slices
- 1 cup mozzarella cheese
- 1 cup olives

DIRECTIONS

1. Spread tomato sauce on the pizza crust
2. Place all the toppings on the pizza crust
3. Bake the pizza at 425 F for 12-15 minutes

4. When ready remove pizza from the oven and
    serve

Serves: *4*

Prep Time: *10*   Minutes

Cook Time: *20*   Minutes

Total Time: *30*   Minutes

INGREDIENTS

- 1 tablespoon olive oil
- 1 lb. cauliflower
- ¼ red onion
- ½ cup all-purpose flour
- ¼ tsp salt
- ¼ tsp pepper
- 1 can vegetable broth
- 1 cup heavy cream

DIRECTIONS

1. In a saucepan heat olive oil and sauté cauliflower until tender
2. Add remaining ingredients to the saucepan and bring to a boil

3. When all the vegetables are tender transfer to a blender and blend until smooth

4. Pour soup into bowls, garnish with parsley and serve

Serves: *4*

Prep Time: *10*   Minutes

Cook Time: *20*   Minutes

Total Time: *30*   Minutes

INGREDIENTS

- 1 tablespoon olive oil
- 1 lb. zucchini
- 2 tablespoons garlic
- ¼ red onion
- ½ cup all-purpose flour
- ¼ tsp salt
- ¼ tsp pepper
- 1 can vegetable broth
- 1 cup heavy cream

DIRECTIONS

1. **In a saucepan heat olive oil and sauté garlic until tender**

2. Add remaining ingredients to the saucepan and
    bring to a boil

3. When all the vegetables are tender transfer to a
    blender and blend until smooth

4. Pour soup into bowls, garnish with parsley and
    serve

Serves: *4*

Prep Time: *10*   Minutes

Cook Time: *20*   Minutes

Total Time: *30*   Minutes

INGREDIENTS

- 1 tablespoon olive oil
- 1 lb. spinach
- ¼ red onion
- ½ cup all-purpose flour
- ¼ tsp salt
- ¼ tsp pepper
- 1 can vegetable broth
- 1 cup heavy cream
- 2 leeks

DIRECTIONS

1. In a saucepan heat olive oil and sauté leek until tender

2. Add remaining ingredients to the saucepan and bring to a boil

3. When all the vegetables are tender transfer to a blender and blend until smooth

4. Pour soup into bowls, garnish with parsley and serve

Serves: *4*

Prep Time: *10*   Minutes

Cook Time: *20*   Minutes

Total Time: *30*   Minutes

INGREDIENTS

- 1 tablespoon olive oil
- 1 lb. carrots
- ¼ red onion
- ½ cup all-purpose flour
- ¼ tsp salt
- ¼ tsp pepper
- 1 can vegetable broth
- 1 cup heavy cream

DIRECTIONS

1. In a saucepan heat olive oil and sauté carrots until tender

2. Add remaining ingredients to the saucepan and bring to a boil

3. When all the vegetables are tender transfer to a blender and blend until smooth

4. Pour soup into bowls, garnish with parsley and serve

Serves: **4**

Prep Time: **10**   Minutes

Cook Time: **20**   Minutes

Total Time: **30**   Minutes

INGREDIENTS

- 1 tablespoon olive oil
- ¼ red onion
- ½ cup all-purpose flour
- ¼ tsp salt
- ¼ tsp pepper
- 1 can vegetable broth
- 1 cup heavy cream
- 1 cup celery

DIRECTIONS

1. **In a saucepan heat olive oil and sauté onion until tender**
2. **Add remaining ingredients to the saucepan and bring to a boil**

3. When all the vegetables are tender transfer to a blender and blend until smooth

4. Pour soup into bowls, garnish with parsley and serve

Serves: **2**

Prep Time: **10**   Minutes

Cook Time: **20**   Minutes

Total Time: **30**   Minutes

INGREDIENTS

- ½ lb. asparagus
- 1 tablespoon olive oil
- ½ red onion
- 2 eggs
- ¼ tsp salt
- 2 oz. cheddar cheese
- 1 garlic clove
- ¼ tsp dill

DIRECTIONS

1. In a bowl whisk eggs with salt and cheese
2. In a frying pan heat olive oil and pour egg mixture

3. Add remaining ingredients and mix well
4. Serve when ready

Serves: **2**
Prep Time: **10** Minutes

Cook Time: **20** Minutes

Total Time: **30** Minutes

INGREDIENTS

- ½ lb. spinach
- 1 tablespoon olive oil
- ½ red onion
- ¼ tsp salt
- 2 eggs
- 2 oz. cheddar cheese
- 1 garlic clove
- ¼ cup corn
- ¼ tsp dill

DIRECTIONS

1. In a bowl whisk eggs with salt and cheese

2. In a frying pan heat olive oil and pour egg
    mixture

3. Add remaining ingredients and mix well

4. Serve when ready

Serves: **2**

Prep Time: **10** Minutes

Cook Time: **20** Minutes

Total Time: **30** Minutes

INGREDIENTS

- 1 cup edamame
- 1 tablespoon olive oil
- ½ red onion
- 2 eggs
- ¼ tsp salt
- 2 oz. cheddar cheese
- 1 garlic clove
- ¼ tsp dill

DIRECTIONS

1. In a bowl whisk eggs with salt and cheese
2. In a frying pan heat olive oil and pour egg mixture

3. Add remaining ingredients and mix well

4. Serve when ready

Serves: *2*

Prep Time: *10*   Minutes

Cook Time: *20*   Minutes

Total Time: *30*   Minutes

INGREDIENTS

- 8-10 slices prosciutto
- 1 tablespoon olive oil
- ½ red onion
- ¼ tsp salt
- 2 eggs
- 2 oz. parmesan cheese
- 1 garlic clove
- ¼ tsp dill

DIRECTIONS

1. **In a bowl whisk eggs with salt and parmesan cheese**
2. **In a frying pan heat olive oil and pour egg mixture**

3. Add remaining ingredients and mix well

4. When prosciutto and eggs are cooked remove
    from heat and serve

Serves: *2*
Prep Time: *10*   Minutes

Cook Time: *20*   Minutes

Total Time: *30*   Minutes

INGREDIENTS

- 1 cup eggplant
- 1 tablespoon olive oil
- ½ red onion
- ¼ tsp salt
- 2 eggs
- 2 oz. cheddar cheese
- 1 garlic clove
- ¼ tsp dill

DIRECTIONS

1. In a bowl whisk eggs with salt and cheese
2. In a frying pan heat olive oil and pour egg mixture

3. Add remaining ingredients and mix well
4. Serve when ready

Serves: *2*
Prep Time: *10*   Minutes

Cook Time: *30*   Minutes

Total Time: *40*   Minutes

INGREDIENTS

- 1 lb. sweet potatoes
- ¼ tsp garlic powder
- ¼ tsp paprika
- ¼ tsp salt
- ½ cup parmesan

DIRECTIONS

1. Cut potatoes into thick wedges
2. Place them on a baking sheet
3. Sprinkle with seasoning and toss to coat
4. Roast at 400 F for 25-30 minutes or until golden
5. When ready remove from the oven and serve with parmesan cheese

Serves: *4*

Prep Time: *10*   Minutes

Cook Time: *30*   Minutes

Total Time: *40*   Minutes

INGREDIENTS

- 2 cups chickpeas
- 2 tsp olive oil
- 1 tsp salt
- ¼ tsp smoked paprika
- ¼ tsp garlic powder

DIRECTIONS

1. Place the chickpeas on a baking sheet
2. Sprinkle the seasoning over the chickpeas
3. Drizzle olive oil and toss to coat
4. Bake at 400 F for 28-30 minutes or until they are crunchy
5. When ready remove from the oven and serve

Serves: *4-5*
Prep Time: *10*   Minutes

Cook Time: **25**   Minutes

Total Time: **35**   Minutes

INGREDIENTS

- 1 cup mozzarella cheese
- ½ cup cheddar cheese
- ¼ cup parmesan cheese
- 1 cup ham
- 3-4 eggs

DIRECTIONS

1. In a bowl whisk the eggs with mozzarella cheese, cheddar cheese and parmesan cheese
2. Stir in diced ham
3. Divide the mixture into 4-5 portions and form round rolls
4. Place them on a baking sheet
5. Bake at 350 F for 22-25 minutes

6. When ready remove from the oven and serve

Serves: *4*

Prep Time: *10*   Minutes

Cook Time: *20*   Minutes

Total Time: *30*   Minutes

INGREDIENTS

- 4 salmon fillets
- 1 tablespoon butter
- 1 tsp salt
- ¼ tsp pepper
- 1 lemon

DIRECTIONS

1. Place the salmon on a baking sheet
2. Spread melted butter over the salmon
3. Sprinkle with salmon and pepper
4. Spread lemon slices over the salmon filet
5. Bake at 400 F for 18-20 minutes
6. When ready remove from the oven and serve

Serves: **2**
Prep Time: **10**   Minutes

Cook Time: **20**   Minutes

Total Time: **30**   Minutes

INGREDIENTS

- 10-12 oz. pasta
- 2 tablespoons butter
- 2 garlic cloves
- 2 tablespoons flour
- 1 cup milk
- ¼ tsp salt
- ¼ tsp pepper

DIRECTIONS

1. Cook pasta al dente
2. In a saucepan add melt butter and add garlic
3. Cook for 2-3 minutes
4. Add flour, milk and bring to a simmer

5. Cook until mixture thickness

6. Add pasta to the sauce, salt, pepper and mix well

7. Serve when ready

Serves: **2**

Prep Time: **5**   Minutes

Cook Time: **5**   Minutes

Total Time: **10**   Minutes

INGREDIENTS

- 1 cup cooked chicken breast
- 1 tablespoon pecans
- 2 tablespoons cranberries
- ¼ cup red onion
- 2 tablespoons Greek yogurt
- 1 tsp dried thyme
- 1 cup salad dressing

DIRECTIONS

1. In a bowl mix all ingredients and mix well
2. Serve with dressing

Serves: **2**

Prep Time: **5**   Minutes

Cook Time: **5**   Minutes

Total Time: **10**   Minutes

INGREDIENTS

- 4 cups romaine lettuce
- 2 pears
- ½ cup cranberries
- ¼ cup pecans
- ¼ cup red onion
- 4 slices turkey bacon
- ¼ cup cheese

DIRECTIONS

1. In a bowl mix all ingredients and mix well
2. Serve with dressing

Serves: **2**
Prep Time: **5**   Minutes

Cook Time: **5**   Minutes

Total Time: **10**   Minutes

INGREDIENTS

- **5 cups watermelon**
- **½ cup feta cheese**
- **¼ red onion**
- **¼ black olives**
- **3 tablespoons rice vinegar**

DIRECTIONS

1. **In a bowl mix all ingredients and mix well**
2. **Serve with dressing**

Serves: **2**

Prep Time: **5**   Minutes

Cook Time: **5**   Minutes

Total Time: **10**   Minutes

INGREDIENTS

- 4 cups white potato
- 1 pinch salt
- 2 tablespoons olive oil
- ¼ cup corn
- ½ cup black beans
- 2 tablespoons lemon juice

DIRECTIONS

1. In a bowl mix all ingredients and mix well
2. Serve with dressing

Serves: **2**

Prep Time: **5**   Minutes

Cook Time: **5**   Minutes

Total Time: **10**   Minutes

INGREDIENTS

- **4 cups cooked white potato**
- **2 tablespoons olive oil**
- **¼ cup red bell pepper**
- **¼ cup red onion**
- **½ cup corn**
- **¼ cup cilantro**
- **1 tsp garlic**
- **1 cup salad dressing**

DIRECTIONS

1. **In a bowl mix all ingredients and mix well**
2. **Serve with dressing**

Serves: **2**

Prep Time: **5**   Minutes

Cook Time: **5**   Minutes

Total Time: **10**   Minutes

INGREDIENTS

- 2 cups watermelon
- ¼ red onion
- ¼ cup fete cheese
- 2 cups tomatoes
- 1 tablespoon basil
- 1 cup salad dressing

DIRECTIONS

1. In a bowl mix all ingredients and mix well
2. Serve with dressing

Serves: **2**
Prep Time: **5**   Minutes

Cook Time: **5**   Minutes

Total Time: **10**   Minutes

INGREDIENTS

- **1 package baby spinach**
- **1 cup cantaloupe**
- **1 cucumber**
- **1 cup red onion**
- **2 tablespoons honey**

DIRECTIONS

1. **In a bowl mix all ingredients and mix well**
2. **Serve with dressing**

Serves: **2**

Prep Time: **5**   Minutes

Cook Time: **5**   Minutes

Total Time: **10**   Minutes

INGREDIENTS

- 3 cups tomatoes
- 2 oz. mozzarella cheese
- 2 tablespoons basil
- 1 tablespoon olive oil

DIRECTIONS

1. In a bowl mix all ingredients and mix well
2. Serve with dressing

Serves: 2
Prep Time: 5   Minutes

Cook Time: 5   Minutes

Total Time: *10* Minutes

INGREDIENTS

- 6 cups greens
- 1 cup strawberries
- 2 kiwis
- 1 tablespoon sesame seeds
- ¼ rice vinegar
- 1 cup salad dressing

DIRECTIONS

1. In a bowl mix all ingredients and mix well
2. Serve with dressing

Serves: **2**

Prep Time: **5**   Minutes

Cook Time: **5**   Minutes

Total Time: **10**   Minutes

INGREDIENTS

- 4 cups kale
- 1 cup red cabbage
- 1 apple
- ¼ red onion
- ½ carrot
- ½ cucumber
- 1 cup salad dressing

DIRECTIONS

1. In a bowl mix all ingredients and mix well
2. Serve with dressing

SIMPLE PIZZA RECIPE

Serves: *6-8*

Prep Time: *10*   Minutes

Cook Time: *15*   Minutes

Total Time: *25*   Minutes

INGREDIENTS

- 1 pizza crust
- ½ cup tomato sauce
- ¼ black pepper
- 1 cup pepperoni slices
- 1 cup mozzarella cheese
- 1 cup olives

DIRECTIONS

1. Spread tomato sauce on the pizza crust
2. Place all the toppings on the pizza crust
3. Bake the pizza at 425 F for 12-15 minutes

4. **When ready remove pizza from the oven and serve**

86

Serves: *6-8*
Prep Time: *10*   Minutes

Cook Time: *15*   Minutes

Total Time: *25*   Minutes

INGREDIENTS

- 1 pizza crust
- ½ cup tomato sauce
- ¼ black pepper
- 1 cup zucchini slices
- 1 cup mozzarella cheese
- 1 cup olives

DIRECTIONS

1. Spread tomato sauce on the pizza crust
2. Place all the toppings on the pizza crust
3. Bake the pizza at 425 F for 12-15 minutes
4. When ready remove pizza from the oven and serve

SUMMER SMOOTHIE

Serves: *1*
Prep Time: *5*   Minutes

Cook Time: *5*   Minutes

Total Time: *10*   Minutes

INGREDIENTS

- ½ cup Greek yogurt
- 2 cups raspberries
- 1 nectarine
- 1 cup ice

DIRECTIONS

1. In a blender place all ingredients and blend until smooth
2. Pour smoothie in a glass and serve

Serves: *1*
Prep Time: *5*   Minutes

Cook Time: *5*   Minutes

Total Time: *10*   Minutes

INGREDIENTS

- 1 cup almond milk
- 1 tablespoon honey
- 1 banana
- 2 cups spinach
- ¼ cucumber

DIRECTIONS

1. In a blender place all ingredients and blend until smooth
2. Pour smoothie in a glass and serve

Serves: *1*
Prep Time: *5*   Minutes

Cook Time: *5*   Minutes

Total Time: *10*   Minutes

INGREDIENTS

- 1 banana
- 1 pineapple
- 1 cup mango
- 1 cup almond milk

DIRECTIONS

1. **In a blender place all ingredients and blend until smooth**
2. **Pour smoothie in a glass and serve**

Serves: *1*

Prep Time: *5*   Minutes

Cook Time: *5*   Minutes

Total Time: *10*   Minutes

INGREDIENTS

- 1 banana
- 4 cups pineapple juice
- 1 cup ice
- 4 oz. blueberries
- 4 oz. blackberries
- 1 tablespoon honey

DIRECTIONS

1. In a blender place all ingredients and blend until smooth
2. Pour smoothie in a glass and serve

Serves: *1*
Prep Time: **5**   Minutes

Cook Time: **5**   Minutes

Total Time: ***10***   Minutes

INGREDIENTS

- 1 cup carrot juice
- 1 banana
- 1 cup pineapple juice
- 1 cup ice

DIRECTIONS

1. **In a blender place all ingredients and blend until smooth**
2. **Pour smoothie in a glass and serve**

Serves: *1*

Prep Time: *5* Minutes

Cook Time: *5* Minutes

Total Time: *10* Minutes

INGREDIENTS

- 1 cup pomegranate juice
- 1 cup yogurt
- 1 cup berries
- 1 cup ice
- 1 cinnamon

DIRECTIONS

1. In a blender place all ingredients and blend until smooth
2. Pour smoothie in a glass and serve

95

Serves: *1*

Prep Time: *5*   Minutes

Cook Time: *5*   Minutes

Total Time: *10*   Minutes

INGREDIENTS

- 1 banana
- 1 cup milk
- 2 tablespoons peanut butter
- 1 cup ice

DIRECTIONS

1. In a blender place all ingredients and blend until smooth
2. Pour smoothie in a glass and serve

Serves: *1*

Prep Time: *5*   Minutes

Cook Time: *5*   Minutes

Total Time: *10*   Minutes

INGREDIENTS

- 1 cup orange juice
- ¼ cup vanilla yogurt
- 1 cup mango
- 1 carrot
- 1 cup ice

DIRECTIONS

1. In a blender place all ingredients and blend until smooth
2. Pour smoothie in a glass and serve

Serves: *1*
Prep Time: **5**   Minutes

Cook Time: **5**   Minutes

Total Time: ***10***   Minutes

INGREDIENTS

- 1 cup strawberries
- ¼ cup blueberries
- 1 cup orange juice
- ½ cup Greek yogurt
- 1 cup ice

DIRECTIONS

1. **In a blender place all ingredients and blend until smooth**
2. **Pour smoothie in a glass and serve**

98

Serves: *1*

Prep Time: *5*   Minutes

Cook Time: *5*   Minutes

Total Time: *10* Minutes

INGREDIENTS

- 1 cup coconut flakes
- ½ cup papaya
- 1 tablespoon goji berries
- 1 tablespoon chia seeds
- 1 banana
- 1 cup ice

DIRECTIONS

1. In a blender place all ingredients and blend until smooth
2. Pour smoothie in a glass and serve

99

THANK YOU FOR READING THIS BOOK!

www.ingramcontent.com/pod-product-compliance
Lightning Source LLC
Chambersburg PA
CBHW051210250726
48655CB00006B/2331